The Blue Zone (

Vegetarian Recipes

Author

Kayla W. Fike

Table of Contents

Consume foods that are high in blue. Meat should be avoided Avoid overindulging.

Reduced calorie intake and fasting are also common among the Blue Zones' habits. Restriction on Calories

Fasting

Alcoholism in moderation Exercise

A good night's sleep and plenty of rest

Meal Plan for Blue Zone Diet Menu from the Blue Zone Diet Tuesdays, Wednesdays, Thursdays, Fridays, Saturdays, and Sundays are the days

Foods to Avoid in the Blue Zones Diet Grains, whole

Beans are a common grain used in recipes.

Nuts are a common ingredient in bean recipes.

Leafy Greens is a popular nut recipe.

Healthy Lifestyle: Popular Leafy Green Recipes In the Blue Zones, there are a variety of practices that are used. Later in the day, eat your smallest meal; when you're only 80% full, stop eating. Stress Reduction

Spend time with friends and family while remaining active. Benefits of a Blue Zone Diet Knowing Your Purpose

It encourages people to interact with one another:

It is environmentally friendly:

You can still have a glass of wine if you follow these guidelines:

There's a lot of fiber in it:

There's no need to eat or drink any weird diet foods or drinks: Section 2:

Vegetarian recipes from the Blue Zones cookbook Vegetarian Blue Flame Blue Angel Blue Flame Blue Angel Blue Flame Blue Angel Blue Flame Blue Angel Blue Flame Cookies in the shape of a strawberry sundae from Sancocho Cookies with Strawberries

Cheesecake with Strawberry Bars with lemon Salad Two Blue Times

Pasta Salad with Strawberry-Asparagus

Slaw with Honey Yogurt Dressing made with Brussels Sprouts Blue Cheese and Grilled Radicchio

Belgian Endive au Gratin Italian-Style: Roasted Lettuce, Radicchio, and Endive Chard de Suisse

Edible Bowl for Spring Pea Medley Salad Dressing: Tahini, Spinach, and Blue Cheese

Dressing with Alaine's blue cheese Blue Cheese Dressing made with buttermilk Bluetons Bluetons Bluetons Bluetons Bluetons Blue (Blue Cheese Croutons) Olive Croutons are the best croutons you will ever have.

Croutons with Garlic & Parmesan Garlic of the Year Croutons with Parmesan Croutons made from an old hamburger bun Croutons made from a croissant

Croutons of Focaccia

Arugula and Watermelon Salad Watermelon and Blue Cheese Salad Herb Watermelon Feta Salad

Introduction

Do you want to live the healthiest, longest life you can? People do it in five places around the world, and one thing they all have in common is how they eat. The populations in these pockets of the planet, dubbed Blue Zones by Dan Buettner, who studies these locales, have an extremely high percentage of nonagenarians and centenarians, respectively, who live to be over 90 and 100 years old. Diabetes, heart disease, cancer, and obesity are all rare in this population.

Overall, the Blue Zones diet resembles other modern diets aimed at reducing chronic disease and improving overall health, such as the Planetary Diet and The OMD Plan, which Oprah recently featured on her SuperSoul Sunday. It's also backed by science and promotes healthy, long-term weight loss as well as overall wellness.

Some of the world's oldest and healthiest people can be found in the Blue Zone regions.

They eat a plant-based diet, exercise regularly, drink moderate amounts of alcohol, get enough sleep, and have strong spiritual, family, and social networks, despite minor differences in their lifestyles. Almost everyone is born with a sweet tooth and a dislike for bitter flavors. This is because sweetness generally denotes calories, whereas bitterness denotes toxins in some cases. Those who ate honey and berries were more likely to survive than those who ate bitter-tasting plants, including greens, which provide vitamins, minerals, and fiber and are a staple of the Blue Zones diet today.

Each of these factors has been linked to a longer life expectancy.

You might be able to add a few years to your life by incorporating them into your daily routine.

What Are Blue Zones? (Chapter 1)

The term "Blue Zone" refers to geographical areas where some of the world's oldest people reside. Surprisingly, only 20–30% of longevity is likely due to genetics. As a result, factors such as diet and lifestyle play a significant role in determining your lifespan.

One thing that all Blue Zone residents have in common is that they eat a plant-based diet that is 95% of the time.

Despite the fact that the majority of the groups are not strict vegetarians, they only eat meat about five times per month. A number of studies, including one involving more than half a million people, have found that avoiding meat lowers the risk of death from heart disease, cancer, and a variety of other causes. Instead, the Blue Zones' diets are typically high in:

Vegetables

They're high in fiber as well as a variety of vitamins and minerals. More than five servings of fruits and vegetables per day can help you avoid heart disease, cancer, and death.

Legumes

Beans, peas, lentils, and chickpeas are all high in fiber and protein, and they're all legumes. Eating legumes has been linked to a lower mortality rate in a number of studies.

Grain, whole

Fiber can also be found in whole grains. Consumption of whole grains is linked to a lower risk of colorectal cancer and heart disease death.

Nuts are high in fiber, protein, and polyunsaturated and monounsaturated fats, among other nutrients. They're linked to lower mortality and may even aid in the reversal of metabolic syndrome when combined with a healthy diet.

Things to stay away from snacks high in sodium

Almost all chips and crackers contain high amounts of salt, preservatives, and highly processed grains, all of which quickly convert to sugar. They've also been meticulously crafted to be crisp and tasty, with a sultry mouthfeel. They're designed to be irresistible, in other words.

Beverages with Added Sugar

Would you ever smother your cereal with ten teaspoons of sugar? No, I doubt it. When you drink a 12-ounce can of soda pop, however, you consume that much sugar on average.

Meats That Have Been Processed

Over half a million people were tracked for decades in a recent gold-standard epidemiology study.

and discovered that people who ate a lot of sausages, salami, bacon, lunch meats, and other highly processed meats had the highest cancer and heart disease rates. The danger is twofold in this case, as well. These meat products contain known carcinogens such as nitrates and other preservatives. They do the job, though, and the products are well preserved, which means that processed meats are readily available on the shelf at home or in the store, ready for snacking or a quick meal, which is not the case in Blue Zones households and diets.

Sweets in a box

Cookies, candy bars, muffins, granola bars, and even energy bars all contain insulin-spiking sugars, just like salty snacks. We're all genetically pre-programmed to crave sweets, so when we get a craving, we instinctively reach for a package of cookies and dig in.

The Blue Zones' Common Dietary Practices Due to the emphasis on whole grains, fruits, vegetables, legumes, nuts, and seeds in plant-based diets, they tend to be higher in fiber. This is significant because high-fiber diets are linked to a variety of health benefits, including.

a gut microbiome that is both healthier and more diverse Body weight must bc rcduced.

Type 2 diabetes risk is lower. Heart attack risk is lower.

Colorectal cancer risks are reduced.

People in the Blue Zones eat a wide variety of plant foods, so their diets are likely higher in fiber than people who eat a Western diet. Another way their diets help them stay healthy is by lowering their cholesterol levels.

Obesity raises the risk of diabetes, heart disease, certain cancers, and other illnesses.

Plant-based diets may help people live longer by reducing their chances of becoming obese.

Large observational studies suggest that eating more animal foods raises BMI and that eating a plant-based diet lowers the risk of gaining weight over time.

Antioxidants

Antioxidants are chemicals found in foods that help prevent cell damage.

Antioxidant-rich diets have been shown to help prevent and reverse chronic diseases such as cancer and heart disease in numerous studies.

Plant foods, such as fruits and vegetables, contain more antioxidants than meat and other animal products, suggesting that plant-based diets, such as those followed by the Blue Zones, may help to reduce disease risk.

Antioxidants are available in a variety of forms. One common practice, however, can be found in four of the five countries.

Blue Zones promotes the consumption of a specific type of antioxidant that is thought to reduce disease and death risk.

While Seventh-day Adventists have a tradition of abstaining from alcohol, many adults in the other Blue Zones regularly consume red wine. Polyphenols, a type of antioxidant found in red wine, have been shown to reduce the risk of cancer, cardiovascular disease, and premature death in studies.

In this way, the Blue Zones diet resembles the Mediterranean Diet, which encourages the consumption of small amounts of red wine with meals.

There are, of course, a few stipulations. Experts currently agree that there is no compelling reason to begin drinking wine if you haven't done so already. Wine consumption should be limited to 1-2 glasses per day for those who already consume alcohol, always with food and ideally with friends or family. Remember that wine, or antioxidants in general, will not compensate for a poor diet. Wine should therefore be paired with a diet high in fruits, vegetables, whole grains, legumes, nuts, seeds, and healthy fats.

Sources of Protein:

Animal proteins contain more saturated fats and cholesterol than plant proteins in general. By incorporating fewer animal proteins and more plant proteins, the Blue Zones Diet could help people live longer.

Those who got the most protein from meat were significantly more likely to die from cardiovascular disease than those who got the most protein from nuts and seeds, according to a study involving more than 81,000 adults.

Other large studies have linked increased meat consumption to an increased risk of death, especially in people with a history of type 2 diabetes, cardiovascular disease, or cancer. Plant-based diets, on the other hand, are associated with a lower risk of death. The mortality risk of meat eaters versus plant eaters was compared in a large study of over 131,000 adults. Replacing 3% of animal protein calories with 3% of plant protein calories resulted in a 10% lower risk of death in this study.

Furthermore, the effect was cumulative, meaning that people who replaced 15% of their animal protein calories with equal amounts of plant protein had a 50% lower risk of death.

To put it another way, even if you're not ready to go vegetarian, you might be able to reduce your disease risk by simply eating less meat.

A Healthy Eating Plan That Could Help You Live Longer Plants account for 95% of your daily diet.

Four of the five Blue Zones eat meat, but only in small amounts. Meat is consumed about five times a month on average, in portions of two ounces or less (think half of a deck of cards). Meat is considered a celebratory food or a way to flavor primarily plant-based dishes, rather than taking up the center of the plate.

In addition to pulses (beans, lentils, peas, chickpeas), fruit, whole grains, nuts, and seeds, residents of the Blue Zone consume a wide variety of vegetables. a half-cup of cooked beans and two tablespoons of olive oil

In the Blue Zones, one ounce of nuts is consumed every day. Furthermore, rather than processed foods, the emphasis is on naturally nutrient-dense whole foods.

Dairy and eggs should be avoided.

Cow's milk products aren't present in significant quantities in four of the five Blue Zones. Goat and sheep milk products are popular in Ikaria and Sardinia. And, rather than eating eggs as a main protein source, people in all of the Blue Zones eat them two to four times a week, usually one at a time and incorporated into a dish. Consider nut-based "cheeses" and plant-based "milks" or "yogurts" as dairy-free alternatives. Consider using eggs as a garnish rather than a main course.

Sugar should be minimized.

Blue Zone residents consume about a fifth of what North Americans do in terms of added sugar per day. The amounts are comparable to the American Heart Association's recommendations, which limit added sugar to six teaspoons per day for women and nine teaspoons per day for men. Sugar is also consumed as a reward by Blue Zone residents. It's not in processed foods, and it's not something you eat out of habit.

Consider a different beverage.

Water, coffee, tea, and wine are the only beverages consumed by people in the Blue Zones, with few exceptions. Every day, tea is sipped in all five Blue Zones, and most people drink one to three small glasses of red wine. Replace soda with H2O or unsweetened tea instead of regular or diet soda. Replace carb-laden beer and sugary mixed drinks with antioxidant-rich red wine as part of a healthy meal.

Water

They cite research showing that staying hydrated improves blood flow and reduces the risk of a blood clot. There is an additional benefit, in my opinion: People who drink water aren't drinking sugary beverages (soda, energy drinks, and fruit juices) or artificially sweetened beverages, many of which are potentially carcinogenic.

coffee

Coffee consumption has been linked to a reduced risk of dementia and Parkinson's disease, according to research. Furthermore, coffee is commonly grown in the shade in the world's blue zones, which benefits birds and the environment.

Tea

Green tea has been shown to reduce the risk of heart disease and several cancers, and it is consumed by people in all of the blue zones.

Wine (red)

The majority of blue zone residents drink one to three glasses of red wine per day, usually with a meal and with friends. Wine has been shown to aid the body's absorption of plant-based antioxidants, making it an excellent addition to the Blue Zones diet. These advantages could be attributed to resveratrol, a red wine antioxidant. However, it's possible that a glass of wine at the end of the day helps to relieve stress, which is beneficial to overall health. More than two to three glasses per day, in any case.

Both women and men suffer from negative health consequences. Women who drink more than one drink per day have a higher risk of breast cancer.

Beans: A Daily Dose

A half cup of cooked beans should be consumed every day.

In the Blue Zones diet, beans are the ultimate superfood. They contain 21% protein, 77 percent complex carbohydrates (the kind that provide a slow and steady energy rather than the spike you get from refined carbohydrates like white flour), and only a few percent fat on average. They're high in fiber, too. They're inexpensive and adaptable, with a variety of textures and more nutrients per gram than any other food on the planet.

Fish should be limited (if you eat it)

People in most Blue Zones consume three small servings of fish per week. However, they are typically middle-of-the-food-chain species (like sardines, anchovies, and cod) that are not exposed to high levels of mercury or other harmful chemicals. Blue Zone societies also don't overfish their waters, and they focus on food sustainability. If you eat seafood, take advantage of a resource like the Environmental Working Group's seafood guide. The free chart they provide rates seafood options using a green, yellow, and red system, based on mercury content and sustainability. Stick with green choices for the greatest benefits, in three ounce portions, up to three times a week.

Sour on Bread\sReplace common bread with sourdough or 100 percent whole wheat bread.

Refined flour is not the only problem inherent to our customary white or wheat breads. Gluten, a protein, gives bread its loft and texture, but it also creates digestive problems for some people. Bread in the Blue Zones diet is different: either whole grain or sourdough, each with its own healthful characteristics. Breads in Ikaria and Sardinia, for example, are made from a variety of 100 percent whole grains, including wheat, rye, and barley each of which offer a wide spectrum of nutrients, such as tryptophan, an amino acid, and the minerals selenium and magnesium.

Consume foods that are high in blue.

Integrate at least three of these items into your daily Blue Zones diet to be sure you are eating plenty of whole food.

Beans—all kinds: black beans, pinto beans, garbanzo beans, black eyed peas, lentils Greens—spinach, kale, chards, beet tops, fennel tops

Sweet potatoes—don't confuse with yams

Nuts—all kinds: almonds, peanuts, walnuts, sunflower seeds, Brazil nuts, cashews

Olive oil—green, extra-virgin is usually the best. (Note that olive oil decomposes quickly, so buy no more than a month's supply at a time.)

Oats—slow-cooking or Irish steel cut are best

Barley—either in soups, as a hot cereal, or ground in bread Fruits—all kinds

Green or herbal teas Turmeric- as a spice or a tea

Retreat from Meat

Consume meat no more than twice a week.

Eat meat twice a week or even less in servings sized no more than two ounces cooked. Favor true free-range chicken and family-farmed pork or lamb instead of meats raised industrially. Avoid processed meats like hot dogs, luncheon meats, or sausages.

In most Blue Zones diets people ate small amounts of pork, chicken, or lamb. (Adventists, the one exception, ate no meat at all.) Families traditionally slaughtered their pig or goat for festival celebrations, ate heartily, and preserved the leftovers, which they would then use sparingly as fat for frying or as a condiment for flavor. Chickens roamed on the land, eating grubs and roosting freely. But chicken meat, likewise, was a rare treat savored over many meals. Averaging out meat consumption over all Blue Zones, we found that people were eating small amounts of meat, about two ounces or less at a time, about five times per month. About once a month they splurged, usually on roasted pig or goat. Neither beef nor turkey figures significantly into the average Blue Zones diet.Take care not to overeat.

Overeating is not a problem in the Blue Zone. They also eat mostly home-cooked meals, with breakfast being the most important and dinner being the least important. Slow down your food consumption. Between bites, put your utensil down, pay attention to your inner fullness meter, and stop when you're satisfied. Also, "front load" your eating pattern by shifting the majority of your intake to the morning, when you're more active. A larger breakfast, such as a veggie, bean, and avocado scramble with a side of fresh fruit, and a lighter dinner, such as a salad with an extra virgin olive oil vinaigrette and a cup of lentil soup, are both good choices.

Reduced calorie intake and fasting are two other Blue Zone habits. Calorie Restriction is a diet that restricts the amount of calories consumed.

Calorie restriction for a long period of time could help you live longer.

In a 25-year study of monkeys, researchers discovered that eating 30% fewer calories than usual resulted in significantly longer life.

Some of the Blue Zones' residents may live longer because they consume fewer calories. This keeps them from overeating, which can lead to obesity and chronic disease.

Eating slowly, as opposed to eating quickly, has been shown in a number of studies to reduce hunger and increase feelings of fullness.

This could be due to the fact that the hormones that make you feel full reach their peak blood levels 20 minutes after you eat.

As a result, you can eat fewer calories and feel fuller for longer by eating slowly and only until you feel 80% full.

Fasting

Periodic fasting appears to be beneficial to health in addition to consistently reducing overall calorie intake. In humans, many other types of fasting have been shown to lower weight, blood pressure, cholesterol, and a variety of other chronic disease risk factors. Fasting mimicking, which involves fasting for a few consecutive days per month, and intermittent fasting, which involves fasting for certain hours of the day or certain days of the week.

Drinking alcohol in moderation

Moderate alcohol consumption is another dietary characteristic shared by many Blue Zones.

The evidence on whether moderate alcohol consumption lowers the risk of death is conflicting.

Many studies have shown that drinking one to two alcoholic drinks per day reduces mortality, particularly from heart disease.

However, when other lifestyle factors are taken into account, a recent study suggests that there is no real effect.

Moderate alcohol consumption may have different effects depending on the type of alcohol consumed. Given that red wine contains many antioxidants derived from grapes, it may be the best type of alcohol.

Antioxidants protect DNA from damage, which can speed up the aging process. As a result, antioxidants may play a role in extending one's lifespan. Drinking moderate amounts of red wine has been linked to a slightly longer life span in several studies. However, as with other alcohol studies, it's unclear whether this effect is due to wine drinkers' healthier lifestyles. People who drank a 5-ounce (150-ml) glass of wine every day for six months to two years had significantly lower blood pressure, blood sugar, more "good" cholesterol, and improved sleep quality, according to other studies. It's important to note that these advantages are only seen when drinking in moderation. Higher levels of consumption, according to each of these studies, increase the risk of death.

Exercise is another important factor in aging, in addition to diet.

People in the Blue Zones do not go to the gym with the intention of exercising. Instead, gardening, walking, cooking, and other daily chores are woven into their lives.

A study of over 13,000 men previously demonstrated the benefits of these routine activities. Every day, the distance they walked or the number of stories of stairs they climbed predicted how long they would live. Exercise has also been shown to lower the risk of cancer, heart disease, and death in other studies. Physical Activity Guidelines for Americans currently recommend a minimum of 75 minutes of vigorous-intensity or 150 minutes of moderate-intensity aerobic activity per week.

According to a large study involving over 600,000 people, those who exercised the recommended amount had a 20% lower risk of dying than those who did not.

Increasing your physical activity can lower your risk of death by up to 39%.

Another large study found that vigorous exercise reduced the risk of death compared to moderate exercise.

A good night's sleep and enough rest

Aside from exercise, getting enough rest and getting a good night's sleep appears to be very important.

vital to a long and healthy life

Blue Zone residents get enough sleep and frequently nap during the day.

Several studies have discovered that not getting enough sleep, or sleeping too much, increases the risk of death from heart disease or stroke.

Seven hours of sleep was found to be the optimal sleep duration in a large review of 35 studies. Sleeping significantly less or significantly more than that was linked to a higher risk of death. People in the Blue Zones don't go to bed, wake up, or work at regular times. They simply sleep for as long as their bodies require.

Daytime naps, known as "siestas" in many Mediterranean countries, have been shown in a number of studies to have no negative impact on the risk of heart disease and death, and may even lower these risks.

The length of the nap, on the other hand, seems to be crucial. 30 minute naps may be beneficial, but anything more than that is linked to an increased risk of heart disease and death.

Meal Plan for The Blue Zone Diet A Sample Menu for the Blue Zone Diet

There are breakfast, lunch, and dinner recipes in the meal plan.

Monday: Banana Yogurt Pots Lunch: Cannellini Bean Salad Quick Moussaka for Dinner

Tomato and Watermelon Salad (Tuesday Breakfast) Veggie Wraps with a Kick

Spicy Baked Eggs with Tomatoes

Wednesday

Dinner: Salmon with Potatoes and Corn Salad Breakfast: Blueberry Oats Bowl Lunch: Carrot, Orange, and Avocado Salad Dinner: Salmon with Potatoes and Corn Salad Thursday: Banana Yogurt Pots for Breakfast, Mixed Bean Salad for Lunch, and Spiced Carrot and Lentil Soup for Dinner

Tomato-Watermelon Salad for Breakfast Dinner-Med Chicken, Quinoa, and Greek Salad Lunch- Panzanella Salad

Saturday

Blueberry Oats Bowl for breakfast; Quinoa and Stir-Fried Veggies for lunch

Dinner: Bean Mash with Grilled Vegetables

Sunday

Banana Yogurt Pots for breakfast Dinner-Spicy Mediterranean Beet Salad Lunch- Moroccan Chickpea Soup

Food Recommendations for the Blue Zones Diet Grain (whole)

The Blue Zones Diet recommends eating whole grains such as farro, quinoa, brown rice, oatmeal bulgur, and cornmeal. Fiber-rich and extremely filling, these grains are a must-try. In comparison to grains made from bleached white flour or processed grains, they are also more likely to release calories as energy rather than stored fat.

Farro with Mushrooms is a popular grain recipe. Steel-Cut Oatmeal with Quinoa Salad

Beans, legumes, and pulses make up the majority of blue zone residents' diets. Blue zone residents consume four times the amount of beans consumed by the average American. They're high in protein, fiber, and complex carbohydrates (the kind that give you long-lasting energy), and they're also inexpensive.

Bean Recipes You'll Love:

Salad II with Black Beans and Corn Healthy Garden Salad with Chickpeas

Nuts should be consumed in two handfuls per day, according to the Blue Zones Diet's food guidelines. They discovered that people who eat nuts live an average of 2 to 3 years longer than those who don't. Almonds, peanuts, Brazil nuts, cashews, and walnuts are all high in important nutrients and make up the ideal nut mix.

Terrific Trail Mix is a popular nut recipe. Trail Mix Full of Antioxidants

Almond 'You've GOT TO BE KIDDING ME!' Crackers

Greens, Leafy

What, according to the Blue Zones Diet, is the best of all longevity foods? Greens with lots of leaves Spinach, kale, beet and turnip tops, chard, and collards are some of the vegetables that fall into this category. Vitamins A and C, for example, have strong antioxidant properties.

Mediterranean Kale is a popular leafy green.

Salad with cranberries and spinach, prepared by Jamie Oliver Soup with Lentils and Collards

In the Blue Zones, Healthy Lifestyle Practices

In the Blue Zones and elsewhere, a balanced diet is essential for long life and good health.

Optimal health, on the other hand, necessitates more than just a nutritious diet. Blue Zone residents share a set of lifestyle habits that complement their healthy eating habits. Here are some suggestions to get you started.

Later in the day, consume your smallest meal.

"Eat breakfast like a king, lunch like a prince, and dinner like a pauper," goes the saying.

This eating pattern is prevalent in the Blue Zones, and it may be beneficial to their health. Indeed, large observational studies have linked large evening meals and late-night snacking to an increased risk of obesity, metabolic syndrome, and other health problems.

When you are only 80% full, you should stop eating.

The world's healthiest people eat until they're stuffed. Instead, they eat until they are about 80% full. They eat fewer calories overall as a result, lowering their risk of obesity and obesity-related diseases. When you're used to eating until you're stuffed, it can be difficult to stop eating at the point of satisfaction. Adopting mindful eating practices is the best way to do so. To get you started, here are some suggestions:

All devices should be turned off while you eat at the table. Meals should be taken slowly and thoroughly chewed.

Take a quick break if you're not sure if you're at least 80% full. If you still feel hungry, you can always have more.

Control your anxiety.

Prayer, meditation, and naps are just a few of the ways people in the Blue Zones manage their stress every day. They may be able to reduce the risk of inflammation and cardiovascular disease as a result of their efforts.

Make a list of activities that bring you joy and peace, such as going for a long walk or talking on the phone with a friend.

A hot bath, a friend, or meditation are all good ideas. Making time for these activities can help you prevent stress from occurring in the first place, as well as make you feel more calm when you do.

Keep yourself busy.

Blue Zone residents are physically active but do not necessarily "work out."

Their communities, on the other hand, promote activity in subtle ways. Blue Zone residents prefer to walk or bike rather than drive, and they don't mind doing manual labor around the house or in the garden. One of the reasons they live longer than people in other parts of the world is because of this.

Spend Quality Time with Family and Friends

People in the Blue Zones place a high value on spending time with friends and family, and they may live longer as a result.

Making time for important people in your life, no matter how busy you are, is essential. Try taking a class, joining a senior center, or volunteering if you want to expand your social circle.

Be aware of your goal.

A meta-analysis involving ten studies and over 136,000 participants discovered significant links between having a clear sense of purpose in life and a reduced risk of death from any cause.

The Blue Zone's Advantages Diet

The Blue Zones plan has benefits and drawbacks like any other diet, but the benefits outweigh the drawbacks. The following is a list of the various advantages:

It encourages socialization:

Many other diets have strict eating windows or restrict the types of food you can eat, making eating with others nearly impossible. The Blue Zones Diet promotes social eating and drinking, making it more enjoyable than other diets.

It is beneficial to the environment:

The Blue Zones Diet is a plant-based diet that is good for both your health and the health of Mother Earth.

You can still drink wine if you want to:

Unlike many other diets, where alcohol is prohibited, if you enjoy a nightly glass of wine, it is still encouraged.

It has a high fiber content:

The foundation of the Blue Zones Diet is beans, vegetables, fruits, nuts, and whole grains, which are also high in soluble and insoluble fiber. Dietary fiber consumption has been linked to weight loss as well as gut and cardiovascular health.

There's no need for wacky diet foods or beverages:

Instead of gimmicky, expensive diet foods or supplements, this diet is based on whole, nutrient-dense foods that are readily available in your local supermarket.

Chapter 2: Vegetarian Recipes from the Blue Zones

Over peppermint schnapps, a layer of Blue Flame Southern Comfort is poured on top. It's then lit, and a blue flame appears. Before you drink, remember to blow it out.

2 mins to prepare 2 mins total 1 serving Southern Comfort 12 fl oz

peppermint schnapps, 12 fluid ounces

Directions 1.

In a small fluted glass, pour the schnapps over ice. Place a teaspoon just above the schnapps and slowly pour Southern Comfort onto it, allowing it to run in a separate layer on top of the schnapps. It has to be layered, not mixed.

Step 2 Light the Southern Comfort with a match or lighter, holding the glass away from your face. Allow for 15 seconds of burning time. It should be blown out and sucked down.

Facts on Nutrition

197 calories per serving; 0 grams of protein; 19.9 grams of carbohydrates; 0.1 grams of fat; 0 milligrams of cholesterol; and 3.1 milligrams of sodium

Angel of the Seas 5 mins to prepare

5 mins total 1 serving

1 oz. brandy, 1 oz. rum

Blue Curacao, 12 fl. oz.

Vanilla liqueur, 12 fluid ounce

half-and-half cream, 12 fluid ounces lemon juice, a dash

1 lemon slice as a finishing touch

Directions 1.

Mix brandy, Blue Curacao, vanilla liqueur, half-and-half, and lemon juice in a cocktail mixer with plenty of ice. Pour into a chilled cocktail glass after a vigorous shake. A lemon slice and a straw are optional garnishes.

Per serving: 212 calories, 0.6 grams of protein, 15.8 grams of carbohydrates, 1.9 grams of fat, 5.6 milligrams of cholesterol, and 8.9 milligrams of sodium

Sancocho de Veggies 30 Minutes to prepare

50 minutes in the oven 1 hr and 20 minutes in total Servings:14 Servings per recipe: 14 Ingredients

2 tbsp.

2 quarts vegetable stock 1 yellow onion chopped

peeled and cut into 1-inch cubes 2 yuca (cassava) roots 2 Yukon Gold potatoes (1-inch cubes)

2 red potatoes (1-inch cubes)

2 peeled plantains, sliced lengthwise into thirds and cut into strips 2 husked and cut-in-thirds ears yellow corn

1 bunch green onions, lemon juiced (chopped)

1 bunch chopped cilantro (divided) 3-garlic cloves

paprika, 14 teaspoon (or to taste)

Step 1: Follow the directions

To taste, season with salt and black pepper. sliced avocados

Over medium-high heat, melt butter in a large pot. 5 minutes later, the onion should be translucent. Bring to a boil with the vegetable stock.

Step 2: Lower the heat to a low setting. In a large pot, combine the yuca, Yukon potatoes, and red potatoes; cook for 15 minutes, or until softened. Cook for 20 minutes, stirring occasionally, until plantains and corn are tender. Combine the green onion, lemon juice, half of the cilantro, garlic, and paprika in a large mixing bowl. Using salt and pepper, season to taste. Cook for 5 minutes, or until all of the flavors are well blended.

3rd Action

Place avocado and the remaining cilantro on top of the soup in serving bowls.

Facts on Nutrition

246 calories per serving; 3.9 grams of protein; 46 grams of carbohydrates; 6.7 grams of fat; 4.4 milligrams of cholesterol; and 305.5 milligrams of sodium

Cookies in the shape of a strawberry sundae

These simple bar cookies taste just like strawberry sundae crunch ice cream bars! Keep refrigerated, covered.

15-minute prep

45-minutes to prepare 2 hr 30 mins additional 3 hr 30 mins in total

Servings:36

36 cookie bars are made from this recipe.

Cooking spray Ingredients

1 strawberry cake mix (15.25 ounces)

12 c. softened butter

softened cream cheese, 2 (8 ounce) packages 1 cream cheese frosting container (16 oz.) 3 oz.

Directions Preheat the oven to 325 degrees Fahrenheit (180 degrees Celsius). Use cooking spray to lightly coat the bottom of a 9x13-inch baking pan.

Step 2 In a large mixing bowl, using an electric mixer on low speed, crumble the cake mix and butter together. 1 cup of the crumble mixture should be set aside; the rest should be pressed into the pan's bottom.

Step 3 In the same bowl, beat the cream cheese and frosting until smooth. In a separate bowl, whisk together the eggs and milk until thoroughly combined. Distribute evenly over the crust. Over the crumble mixture, evenly distribute the remaining crumble mixture.

Step 4 Bake for 45 to 50 minutes in a preheated oven, or until golden brown. Allow 30 minutes for complete cooling. Cover and chill for at least 2 hours.

Step 5: Cut 6x6 rows out of the bars.

If you prefer, you can use margarine instead of butter.

If you prefer, you can make a chocolate version by replacing the strawberry cake mix with chocolate cake mix, or a creamsicle-like version by replacing the strawberry cake mix with orange cake mix.

If you're using a dark or nonstick pan, bake it for a shorter time.

Nutritional Values

176 calories per serving; 1.8 g protein; 17.7 g carbohydrates; 11.2 g fat; 36 mg cholesterol; 166.4 mg sodium

Cake Cookies with Strawberries

Strawberry cake mix and fresh strawberries are used to make these easy strawberry cookies.

Time to prepare: 10 minutes 15 minutes to cook 5 minutes more

30 minutes in total Servings:30 2 1/2 dozen Ingredients

1 package strawberry cake mix (18.25 oz.) 12 cup fresh strawberries, chopped 2 eggs, beaten 1 pound of whipped cream

Directions 1st Step

Preheat the oven to 350°F. Grease cookie sheets with cooking spray.Step 2 In a medium mixing basin, combine the cake mix, eggs, and strawberries until well combined. Fold in the whipped cream until everything is nicely combined. Drop by rounded spoonfuls onto the cookie sheets that have been prepared.

3rd Action

In a preheated oven, bake for 8 to 10 minutes. Allow 5 minutes for cookies to cool on the baking sheet before transferring to a wire rack to cool entirely.

Facts on Nutrition

78 calories per serving; 0.9 g protein; 14.4 g carbs; 2 g fat; 13.9 mg cholesterol; 114.2 mg sodium

Lemon Bars with Strawberry Cheesecake

After supper, treat yourself to lemon cake bars with a strawberry cheesecake filling and a lemon frosting. Refrigerate in an airtight container.

Preparation time: 20 minutes

31 minutes to cook 6 hours and 15 minutes more Total time: 7 hours and 6 minutes Servings:24

24 squares per batch

Cooking spray Ingredients

1 packet (18.25 ounces) lemon cake mix

13 cup lemonade (prepared)

13 cup melted butter

1 (8-ounce) container softened cream cheese

14 cup granulated sugar a single egg

a quarter cup of strawberry preserves

12 CUP CONFECTIONERS' SUCTIONERS' SUCTIONERS'

SUCTIONERS lemon juice, 2 tablespoons

a quarter cup of sprinkles, or to taste

Directions Preheat the oven to 350 degrees Fahrenheit (175 degrees C). Using cooking spray, coat a 9x13-inch baking pan.

Step 2 Combine cake mix, lemonade, and butter in a mixing bowl until a soft dough forms. Half of the dough should be equally distributed in the bottom of the prepared pan.

Step 3 In a mixing basin, beat together cream cheese and sugar until smooth. Add the egg and beat it in again. Cover the dough in the pan with cheesecake.

Step 4 In a microwave-safe dish, combine strawberry preserves. Microwave for 30 seconds, or until completely melted. Drop little spoonfuls of the topping all over the cheesecake layer. To swirl in the strawberry preserves, delicately drag a knifc into the cheesecake.

Step 5 Using the palm of your hand, flatten a tiny portion of the remaining dough. Rip the dough into small pieces and spread over the cheesecake, covering as much as possible.

Step 6 Bake for 30 minutes in a preheated oven until golden brown. Remove from the oven and cool for 2 hours on a wire rack. Refrigerate for 4 hours to overnight until totally cooled.

Step 7 In a mixing dish, combine the confectioners' sugar and lemon juice. Drizzle the mixture over the cold strawberries.

Sprinkle sprinkles on top of the cheesecake. Allow 15 minutes for the frosting to set. Cut the dough into 24 bars.

Tips

Note from the chef: The dough will be sticky at first, but keep pressing until it is uniformly distributed throughout the bottom of the pan. Hands sprayed with nonstick spray are also beneficial.

Facts on Nutrition

187 calories per serving; 2.3 grams of protein; 24.9 grams of carbs; 9 grams of fat; 30.3 milligrams of cholesterol; 203.3 milligrams of sodium

The Times of Blue Salad for two

Blueberries, an antioxidant powerhouse, feature in both the salad and the dressing. With the crumbled blue cheese, the berries create a sweet-tangy combination. They're served with fresh spinach and arugula in a light salad that goes well with grilled meats or roasted chicken.

15-minute prep Total time: 15 minutes Servings:8 8 cup yield Ingredients

4 cups spinach (baby) arugula, 2 cups

12 cup blueberries (about)

12 cup red onion, thinly sliced

13 cup toasted coarsely chopped pecans 14 cup crumbled blue cheese Blue and double blue 1 container (5.3 ounces) VOSKOS® Nonfat Blueberry Greek Yogurt 2 tblsp balsamic vinaigrette

2 tablespoons extra virgin olive oil

2 tblsp blue cheese, crumbled

Directions 1.

In a large mixing dish, combine baby spinach, baby arugula, blueberries, and onion. Dress with the Double Blue Dressing (see below). Toss everything together. Pecans and 1/4 cup blue cheese are sprinkled on top.

2nd Step

In a mixing bowl, combine the VOSKOS® Nonfat Blueberry Greek Yogurt, balsamic vinegar, and olive oil. 2 tablespoons blue cheese, stirred in Refrigerate until ready to serve.

Tips

Preheat the oven to 350 degrees F before toasting the pecans. In a shallow baking pan, spread the pecans and toast for 5 to 10 minutes, stirring the pan once or twice.

Facts on Nutrition

124 calories per serving; 4.3 grams of protein; 8.7 grams of carbs; 8.7 grams of fat; 6 milligrams of cholesterol; 110 milligrams of sodium

Pasta Salad with Strawberry-Asparagus

This vivid side salad with strawberries, asparagus, spinach, and pasta has a creamy dressing made with tangy white balsamic vinegar and VOSKOS® Nonfat Strawberry Greek Yogurt. Serve with grilled steak or roast chicken.

19 minutes to prepare 11 minutes to cook 30 minutes overall Servings:6

There are 6 servings in this recipe. Ingredients

8 oz. penne or bow-tie pasta, uncooked

12 cup asparagus, peeled and chopped into bite-size pieces

2 cups hulled strawberries, quartered lengthwise 12 CUP BABY SPROUTING SPROUTING SPROUTING SPROUT

12 cup goat or feta cheese, crumbled Strawberry-Yogurt 1 container (5.3 ounces) VOSKOS® Nonfat Strawberry Greek Yogurt 2 tblsp balsamic vinegar (white)

2 tablespoons red onion, finely chopped

Directions 1.

Cook the pasta according to package instructions in a large pot, adding the asparagus for the final 2 to 3 minutes or until crisp-tender. Drain the pasta and asparagus, then rinse them with cold water before draining them again. In a large mixing basin, combine all of the ingredients. Toss with the Strawberry Yogurt Dressing (recipe follows).

to amalgamate

2nd Action

Combine the strawberries and spinach in a large mixing bowl and gently fold them in. Sprinkle with goat cheese and transfer to a serving dish.

Step 3: Combine the strawberries and yogurt in a mixing bowl. Dressing: In a large mixing bowl, combine VOSKOS® Nonfat Strawberry Greek Yogurt, balsamic vinegar, and red onion. Refrigerate for up to 24 hours before serving.

Facts on Nutrition

239 calories per serving; 11.3 grams of protein; 38.6 grams of carbs; 4.6 grams of fat; 10.1 milligrams of cholesterol; and 83.9 milligrams of sodium

Slaw with Honey Yogurt Dressing made with Brussels Sprouts

These little heads of cabbage cook quickly in the microwave and slice cleanly for a slaw that combines sweet chopped apple, crumbled bacon, and a creamy Greek yogurt dressing to create a slaw with personality. Brussels sprouts, like other cruciferous vegetables, provide Vitamins A and C, as well as some iron, to the diet.

30 Minutes to prepare

4 minutes to prepare 1 hour 56 minutes additional 2 hour 30 minutes in total Servings:8

8 servings (about)

Ingredients

Brussels sprouts, thinly sliced 1 finely chopped medium apple

4 crisp-cooked and crumbled bacon slices

12 cup toasted sliced almonds yoghurt with honey VOSKOS® Nonfat Honey Greek Yogurt, 1 (5.3 ounce) container 14 teaspoon salt, 1 tablespoon apple cider vinegar

Step 1: Follow the instructions

In a medium microwave-safe dish, combine Brussels sprouts and 2 tablespoons water. Microwave on high for 4 minutes, stirring halfway during the cooking time. Immediately chill the Brussels sprouts by putting them into a dish of cold water and allowing them to drain thoroughly. Use a salad spinner to remove excess moisture from the Brussels sprouts, or set them in a strainer and absorb the moisture with paper towels.

Step 2 In a large mixing basin, toss together the Brussels sprouts and apple. Toss the Brussels sprouts mixture lightly with the Honey Yogurt Dressing (see recipe below). Toss in the bacon and mix gently. Refrigerate for 2–24 hours after covering. Gently toss in almonds just before serving.

In a bowl, combine VOSKOS® Nonfat Honey Greek Yogurt, cider vinegar, and salt. Allow for a 24-hour chilling period.

Tips

Tip 1: To trim Brussels sprouts, snip off the stems right before they begin to produce leaves. Remove the dark green outer leaves until only the fragile, bright green leaves remain.

Preheat the oven to 350°F before toasting the almonds. In a shallow baking pan, spread the almonds out and toast for 5 to 10 minutes, stirring the pan once or twice.

Per serving: 110 calories, 6.8 grams of protein, 9.7 grams of carbs, 5.7 grams of fat, 7.8 milligrams of cholesterol, and 229.5 milligrams of sodium

Blue Cheese with Grilled Radicchio

These vibrant grilled radicchio wedges go well with almost any grilled main dish. The radicchio's inherent sharpness is tempered by the balsamic's sweet, acidic taste and the creamy blue cheese's creamy texture.

10 minute prep ten minutes to prepare 20 minutes total Servings:4 4 servings (about) Ingredients

2 tbsp. white balsamic vinegar 3 tbsp. olive oil

Step 1: Follow the instructions

salt and pepper to taste 12 teaspoon Dijon mustard

radicchio (one head)

2 tbsp. pistachio nuts, finely chopped 2 tbsp. blue cheese, crumbled

Preheat an outside grill to medium heat and brush the grate gently with olive oil.

Step 2 In a small bowl, combine 2 tablespoons extra virgin olive oil, balsamic vinegar, Dijon mustard, salt, and pepper. Discard the dressing.

Step 3: Cut the head of radicchio into four wedges. Drizzle the remaining 1 tablespoon olive oil over the wedges and season gently with salt.

4)

Grill the wedges for 3 to 4 minutes on each side on a preheated grill. Drizzle dressing over the salad and top with pistachios and blue cheese. Right away, serve.

Per serving: 144 calories, 2.5 grams of protein, 4.7 grams of carbs, 13.3 grams of fat, 3.2 milligrams of cholesterol, and 143.4 milligrams of sodium

Endive, radicchio, and roasted lettuce 20 minutes to prepare

ten minutes to prepare 30 minutes overall Servings:6 6 servings (about) 2 half heads of radicchio

2 lengthwise halved Belgian endive heads

1 half head of chicory (curly endive) 1 lengthwise halved head of romaine lettuce

Step 1: Follow the instructions

14 cup pitted Greek olives, 3 tablespoons olive oil, divided

capers, 12 cup

1 tbsp. oregano (dried) 12 tsp. thyme powder 1 teaspoon black pepper, 1 teaspoon salt

1 teaspoon chile powder (dry) (Optional) 2 tbsp Romano cheese (grated) (Optional)

Preheat the oven to 375 degrees Fahrenheit (190 degrees Celsius) (190 degrees C). Preheat the oven to 350°F and grease a baking dish.

Step 2 On the baking sheet, arrange the radicchio, Belgian endive, chicory, and romaine lettuce halves in a single layer. 2 tbsp. extra virgin olive oil

In a small bowl, mix together the olives and capers. In a small mixing bowl, combine oregano, thyme, salt, black pepper, and chile pepper.

Step 4 Using your fingers, stuff interior leaves with olives, capers, and spice mix. To keep stuffing from falling out, tie the halves together with kitchen thread. 1 tablespoon extra virgin olive oil drizzled on top.

Step 5 Bake for 10 to 15 minutes in a preheated oven, or until crisp and wilted. Before serving, remove any kitchen string and top with Romano cheese.

Note from the chef: Radicchio should be long and thin. It is also OK to use the circular type. If you like, you may use escarole instead of chicory endive.

Per serving: 192 calories, 6.3 grams of protein, 16.7 grams of carbs, 12.9 grams of fat, 2.6 milligrams of cholesterol, and 1108.6 milligrams of sodium

Endive Gratin (Belgian Endive)

The ivory-white head of Belgian endive (known as 'witloof' in Dutch or 'chicon' in Belgian French)

with light yellow edges and tightly wrapped leaves, a moderately bitter taste, and a soft juicy mouthfeel

25 minutes to prepare 30 minutes in the oven 55 minutes total Servings:8 8 servings (about) Ingredients

there are eight of them trimmings of Belgian endive 2 tbsp.

2 tblsp flour 1 quart of cream

1 cup Gruyere cheese, grated (distributed) 2 tbsp Parmesan cheese, grated

14 teaspoon ground nutmeg (or to taste) salt and freshly ground black pepper

deli ham, cut into 8 slices

14 cup parsley, chopped

Directions Step 1: Spray a baking dish with nonstick cooking spray.

Step 2 In a large saucepan over medium-high heat, bring a large pot of lightly salted water to a boil. In a large mixing bowl, combine the endives, water, and salt. Cook for 5 to 10 minutes, covered, until vegetables are soft.

Step 3 Melt the butter over medium heat in a saucepan. Stir in the flour until it forms a paste-like consistency and is golden brown in color. Whisk the milk into the flour mixture until it is thick and smooth, stirring continually. 3/4 cup Gruyere cheese, Parmesan cheese, nutmeg, salt, and pepper are mixed in until thoroughly combined. Cook for 10 minutes, stirring often, over medium-low heat.Step 4\sPreheat an oven broiler to low.

Step 5

Drain the endives. Wrap each endive with a slice of ham, and place into the prepared baking dish. Pour the cheese sauce over the endives. Sprinkle with the remaining 1/4 cup Gruyere cheese and parsley.

Step 6

Cook the endives under preheated broiler until cheese is golden brown and sauce bubbles, about 10 minutes.

Facts on Nutrition

Per Serving: 207 calories; protein 12.8g; carbohydrates 20.4g; fat 10.1g; cholesterol 28.7mg; sodium 210.4mg.

Italian-Style Swiss Chard

This recipe for Italian-style Swiss chard has been in the family for years. If you like garlic, this recipe is for you.

10 minute prep 15-minutes to prepare Total:25 mins Servings:4

Yield:4 side dish servings

Ingredients

1 bunch Swiss chard 1 cup water

1 tablespoon salt

olive oil, 2 tablespoons

4 cloves garlic, coarsely chopped

⅛ teaspoon crushed red pepper flakes salt to taste

Directions 1.

Wash the Swiss chard and cut into 1 inch strips. Separate the thick and tough stalk sections from the upper leafy strips.

Step 2\sBring the water and 1 tablespoon of salt to a boil in a large saucepan.

3rd Action

Cook the stalk sections in the salted boiling water for 2 minutes. Stir in the leafy strips and cook until the leaves are wilted and the stalks are fork tender, about 6 minutes. Drain and set aside.

4)

Heat the olive oil, garlic, and red pepper flakes in a large skillet over medium heat until aromatic, about 3 minutes. Add the drained Swiss chard, cook and stir for 2 minutes; season with salt to taste.

Facts on Nutrition

Per Serving: 75 calories; protein 1.2g; carbohydrates 3.2g; fat 6.9g; sodium 1865.7mg.

Edible Bowl for Spring Pea Medley

If you like fresh peas, this is the way to go. It must be done in the Spring with fresh peas. Careful not to get over grown peas, which are woody. Look for smaller peas, and you will LOVE this spring time pea medley. It's BEAUTIFUL, too!

15-minute prep Cook:5 mins 20 minutes total Servings:4 4 servings (about)

Ingredients

2 tbsp.

1 small sweet onion, diced

1 cup fresh shelled green peas

½ cup low sodium, low fat vegetable broth

½ pound sugar snap peas, trimmed

½ pound snow peas, trimmed

1 tablespoon chopped fresh parsley salt and pepper to taste

1 medium head radicchio

Directions 1.

In a medium skillet, melt the butter over medium low heat. Add the onion and saute until transparent, about 5 minutes. Stir in the green peas and the broth, and cook for about 3 minutes. Add the snap peas, snow peas and parsley, and season to taste with salt and pepper. Cook, covered, for about 3 more minutes.

Step 2\sRemove the inner leaves from the radicchio and spread the outer leaves out to make a bowl. Fill the hollow with the pea mixture and garnish with additional Italian parsley.

Nutrition Facts\sPer Serving: 151 calories; protein 5.4g; carbohydrates 18.5g; fat 6.1g; cholesterol 15.3mg; sodium 101.9mg.

Tahini Spinach\sThis is a quick side dish, or mini meal for people who like Middle Eastern flavors!

10 minute prep ten minutes to prepare 20 minutes total Servings:3 Yield:3 servings Ingredients

1 (10 ounce) package frozen chopped spinach

½ cup water

1 tablespoon tahini

2 cloves garlic, minced\s¼ teaspoon ground cumin\s¼ teaspoon paprika

cayenne pepper, or to taste

⅓ cup red wine vinegar salt and pepper to taste

Directions 1.

Place the spinach and water into a saucepan, and bring to a boil over high heat. Reduce heat to medium-low, cover, and simmer 4 to 6 minutes until tender.

Step 2\sMeanwhile, whisk together the tahini, garlic, cumin, paprika, cayenne pepper, and red wine vinegar. Season to taste with salt and pepper. Drain the cooked spinach, and top with the tahini sauce to serve.

Facts on Nutrition

Per Serving: 69 calories; protein 4.5g; carbohydrates 7.8g; fat 3.3g; sodium 77.7mg.

Blue Cheese Salad Dressing

A great salad dressing that can be used anywhere you want to add some extra flavor with blue cheese. Keep refrigerated, covered. Let dressing warm to room temperature and stir with a fork before serving.

10 minute prep Total:10 mins Servings:22 Yield:22 servings Ingredients

4 ounces blue cheese, crumbled 3 tablespoons lemon juice

3 tablespoons tarragon vinegar 2 tablespoons red wine vinegar 2 tablespoons steak sauce

1 tablespoon Worcestershire sauce

1 tablespoon prepared yellow mustard

1 small garlic clove, peeled and chopped

½ teaspoon salt

½ teaspoon ground black pepper 2 cups salad oil

Directions 1.

Combine blue cheese, lemon juice, tarragon vinegar, red wine vinegar, steak sauce, Worcestershire sauce, mustard, garlic, salt, and pepper in a large bowl; beat with an electric mixer until well blended. Gradually mix in salad oil until thoroughly combined. Right away, serve.

Nutrition Facts\sPer Serving: 196 calories; protein 1.2g; carbohydrates 0.8g; fat 21.3g; cholesterol 3.9mg; sodium 160.7mg.

Dressing with Alaine's blue cheese

Once you have tasted this blue cheese dressing recipe, no other will compare. No bottled dressing or restaurant dressing will ever measure up to this killer dressing.

15-minute prep

15 minutes total Servings:20 Yield:20 servings Ingredients\s2 cups mayonnaise

½ pound crumbled blue cheese 1 teaspoon balsamic vinegar

⅛ teaspoon coarsely ground black pepper 1 pinch garlic powder

¼ cup buttermilk

Directions 1.

In a medium bowl, mix mayonnaise, blue cheese, balsamic vinegar, pepper, and garlic powder. Gradually blend in the buttermilk until the dressing has reached the desired consistency. Cover, and refrigerate until serving.

Facts on Nutrition

Per Serving: 200 calories; protein 2.7g; carbohydrates 1.2g; fat 20.8g; cholesterol 17mg; sodium 286.6mg.

Buttermilk Blue Cheese Dressing 5 mins to prepare

Additional:8 hrs Total:8 hrs 5 mins Servings:20 Yield:2 1/2 cups

Ingredients

1 cup buttermilk

1 cup mayonnaise

1 (4 ounce) package crumbled blue cheese

⅛ teaspoon garlic powder

⅛ teaspoon ground black pepper

Step 1: Follow the instructions

Stir the buttermilk, mayonnaise, blue cheese, garlic powder, and black pepper together in a bowl.

2nd Action

Cover bowl with plastic wrap and refrigerate overnight before serving.

Nutrition Facts\sPer Serving: 104 calories; protein 1.7g; carbohydrates 1.1g; fat 10.5g; cholesterol 8.9mg; sodium 154.2mg.

Bluetons Bluetons Bluetons Bluetons Bluetons Blue (Blue Cheese Croutons)

We only use three ingredients here, which is why this works so well. Try to resist the temptation to add salt, pepper, or other spices, as the blue cheese will provide all the punch you need. We're going for pure blue cheese flavor in a buttery, crunchy package, and anything else would just get in the way.

15-minute prep 30 minutes in the oven Total:45 mins Servings:8 8 servings (about) Ingredients

½ loaf fresh bread, cut into 1/2-inch pieces

5 tablespoons unsalted butter, melted and hot, or more to taste 2 ounces frozen blue cheese, grated, or more to taste

Directions 1.

Preheat the oven to 350 degrees Fahrenheit (180 degrees Celsius) (175 degrees C). Line a baking sheet with a silicone baking mat.

Step 2\sPlace bread cubes in a bowl and drizzle butter over the top. Sprinkle about 1/3 of the blue cheese over the top and stir until bread is coated. Sprinkle another 1/3 of the cheese over the top and stir to coat again. Spread bread cubes out onto prepared baking sheet.

3rd Action

Bake in the preheated oven until slightly crisp, about 15 minutes. Toss cubes and sprinkle remaining blue cheese over the top. Bake until browned and crispy, 15 to 20 minutes more.

Nutrition Facts\sPer Serving: 164 calories; protein 3.8g; carbohydrates 14.5g; fat 10.2g; cholesterol 24.4mg; sodium 293.1mg.

Best Croutons Ever\sThese croutons are soft and good.

10 minute prep ten minutes to prepare 20 minutes total Servings:8 Yield:64 croutons Ingredients

¼ cup butter 4 slices bread\s¼ teaspoon garlic powder

Directions 1.

Preheat the oven to 375 degrees Fahrenheit (190 degrees Celsius) (190 degrees C). Line a baking sheet with aluminum foil.

Step 2\sMelt butter in a pot over medium heat.

Step 3\sCut each bread slice into 16 cubes; add bread cubes and garlic powder to melted butter. Stir to coat. Transfer coated bread cubes to the prepared baking sheet.

4)

Bake in the preheated oven until crispy, 8 to 10 minutes.

Facts on Nutrition

Per Serving: 84 calories; protein 1g; carbohydrates 6.4g; fat 6.2g; cholesterol 15.3mg; sodium 126mg.

Olive Croutons 10 minute prep

ten minutes to prepare 20 minutes total Servings:4 4 servings (about)

Ingredients

1 tablespoon extra-virgin olive oil

1 tablespoon tapenade (olive spread) (olive spread) 4 slices ciabatta bread, cut into cubes

Directions 1.

Preheat the oven to 375 degrees Fahrenheit (190 degrees Celsius) (190 degrees C).

Step 2\sStir olive oil and tapenade together in a large bowl; add bread cubes and stir to coat. Spread cubes onto a baking sheet.

3rd Action

Bake in preheated oven until golden brown, 8 to 10 minutes. Cool completely before storing in an airtight container.

Facts on Nutrition

Per Serving: 191 calories; protein 5.1g; carbohydrates 28.7g; fat 6g; cholesterol 0.1mg; sodium 365.1mg.

Croutons with Garlic & Parmesan

These croutons taste great, and your house will smell wonderful with the scent of the herbs.

10 minute prep 15-minutes to prepare Total:25 mins Servings:7 Yield:3 1/2 cups Ingredients

5 tablespoons butter, melted

Step 1: Follow the instructions

1 teaspoon grated Parmesan cheese 1 teaspoon oregano

½ teaspoon dried thyme

½ teaspoon garlic powder

½ teaspoon salt

5 thick slices day-old bread with crusts removed, cut into cubes

Preheat oven to 325 degrees F (165 degrees C).

2nd Action

Mix butter, Parmesan cheese, oregano, thyme, garlic powder, and salt together in a large, flat- bottomed bowl; add bread cubes and turn with a spatula to coat. Spread coated bread cubes onto a baking sheet.

3rd Action

Bake in preheated oven until golden brown, 15 to 20 minutes. Cool croutons completely before storing in an airtight container.

Facts on Nutrition

Per Serving: 133 calories; protein 1.9g; carbohydrates 11.2g; fat 9g; cholesterol 22.1mg; sodium 375.2mg.

Best Garlic Parmesan Croutons

These are like mini garlic bread bites, a perfect addition to caesar salads, soups, or just to munch on! You will never buy another crouton again.

10 minute prep Cook:20 mins 30 minutes overall Servings:8 8 servings (about) Ingredients

8 (1/2 inch thick) slices French bread, cut into 3/4-inch cubes

1 tablespoon creole seasoning (such as Emeril's Bayou Blast!®), or more to taste

½ cup butter

6 tablespoons grated Parmesan cheeseStep 1: Follow the instructions

1 clove garlic, sliced thin ⅛ teaspoon onion powder

Preheat oven to 300 degrees F (150 degrees C).

Step 2 Put cubes in a large bowl and season generously with creole seasoning.

Step 3 Melt butter in a saucepan over medium-low heat. Stir Parmesan cheese, garlic, and onion powder into the melted butter; pour over the bread cubes and toss to coat. Spread bread cubes onto a large baking sheet.

Step 4 Bake in preheated oven for 10 minutes, stir, and continue baking until golden brown and crispy, about 10 minutes more.

Nutrition Facts Per Serving: 193 calories; protein 4.6g; carbohydrates 14.8g; fat 13.1g; cholesterol 33.8mg; sodium 479.4mg.

Old Hamburger Bun Croutons

Have you ever wondered what to do with old extra hamburger buns? Don't throw them away! Turn them into yummy croutons! These are quite tasty, you won't regret making them! This can cater to whatever kind of meal you have. If you want, you can sprinkle Parmesan cheese over them before baking, too.

10 minute prep ten minutes to prepare 20 minutes total Servings:10 Yield:10 servings Ingredients olive oil, or as needed

4 hamburger buns, cut into 1-inch cubes

½ teaspoon garlic powder

Step 1: Follow the instructions

⅛ teaspoon dried oregano

⅛ teaspoon ground thyme

⅛ teaspoon dried basil salt to taste

coarsely ground black pepper to taste

Preheat the oven to 350 degrees Fahrenheit (180 degrees Celsius) (175 degrees C).

2nd Action

Drizzle olive oil over hamburger bun cubs in a large bowl; toss to coat. Spread cubes onto a baking sheet. Sprinkle garlic powder, oregano, thyme, basil, salt, and black pepper over the cubes.

3rd Action

Bake in preheated oven until brown and crispy, 8 to 10 minutes. Cool completely before storing in airtight container.

Cook's Notes:

The oregano, thyme, and basil can be used in whatever proportions you prefer, as long as it's 1/2 teaspoon total.

Store in an airtight container for up to two weeks.

Facts on Nutrition

Per Serving: 62 calories; protcin 1.5g; carbohydrates 8.8g; fat 2.2g; sodium 96.4mg.

Croissant Croutons

Light, airy, and buttery. These croissant croutons are a great way to elevate any simple green salad or tomato soup. Store leftover croutons in and airtight container.

10 minute prep 15-minutes to prepare Total:25 mins Servings:10

Yield:2 1/2 cups croutons

Ingredients

Step 1: Follow the instructions

2 ½ cups croissant cubes, 1-inch wide

⅛ cup olive oil

⅛ cup grated Parmesan cheese ⅛ teaspoon garlic salt

Preheat the oven to 350 degrees F (175 degrees C). Line a baking sheet with parchment paper.

2nd Action

Place croissant cubes in a medium mixing bowl. Drizzle olive oil on top and toss to evenly coat. Stir in Parmesan cheese and garlic salt. Spread croissant cubes evenly on the prepared baking sheet.

3rd Action

Bake in the preheated oven until toasted and light golden brown, 13 to 15 minutes. Let cool to room temperature.

Facts on Nutrition

Per Serving: 64 calories; protein 1.1g; carbohydrates 4.1g; fat 4.8g; cholesterol 6.7mg; sodium 103.1mg.

Croutons of Focaccia

If you've never had freshly made croutons, you might not realize that a crouton doesn't have to just be a rock-hard bread brick that crumbles in your mouth. These from-scratch focaccia croutons are crunchy on the outside but still soft enough in the middle that you can actually chew them.

10 minute prep ten minutes to prepare Additional:40 mins Total:1 hr

Servings:12

Yield:3 1/2 cups croutons

Ingredients

1 clove garlic

¼ cup olive oil

¼ cup grated Parmesan cheese

Step 1: Follow the instructions

⅛ stick butter, melted ½ teaspoon salt

½ teaspoon dried thyme

½ teaspoon onion powder

3 ½ cups rosemary focaccia bread, cut into thumbnail-sized pieces

Crush garlic into a paste with a mortar and pestle.

Step 2 Mix crushed garlic, olive oil, Parmesan cheese, butter, salt, thyme, and onion powder together until relatively homogenous. Let sit for 10 minutes.

Step 3 Place bread cubes in a large bowl and spoon butter mixture on top. Toss well to make sure all the cubes are coated. Cover and let sit until bread soaks up the mixture, about 30 minutes.

Step 4 Preheat the oven to 350 degrees F (175 degrees C). Spread bread on a cookie sheet in a single layer.

Step 5 Bake in the preheated oven, flipping once halfway, until golden brown and firm to the touch, 8 to 10 minutes.

Cook's Note: Make the focaccia from scratch if you really want to go the whole nine yards.

Facts on Nutrition

Per Serving: 80 calories; protein 1.5g; carbohydrates 4.6g; fat 6.2g; cholesterol 4mg; sodium 180.5mg.

Watermelon and Blue Cheese Salad

Refreshing summer salad of watermelon and blue cheese. Great for summer picnics.

20 minutes to prepare 20 minutes total Servings:12

Yield:12 servings

Ingredients

½ cup light olive oil ¼ cup white balsamic vinegar salt and ground black pepper to taste

5 pounds watermelon, cut into bite-size cubes

1 small sweet onion (such as Vidalia®), thinly sliced 2 tablespoons chopped fresh mint, or more to taste

6 ounces crumbled blue cheese

Directions Step 1 Whisk olive oil, vinegar, salt, and pepper together in a bowl until smooth.

Step 2 Mix watermelon, onion, and mint together in a separate bowl. Drizzle dressing over watermelon mixture and add blue cheese; toss well.

Facts on Nutrition

Per Serving: 192 calories; protein 4.3g; carbohydrates 15.9g; fat 13.4g; cholesterol 10.6mg; sodium 201.3mg

Tisa's Big Top Watermelon Salad

Nothing says summer like juicy watermelon. For a unique take on this Fourth of July staple, cube watermelon and toss with feta, onions, pine nuts, and fresh herbs.

20 minutes to prepare 20 minutes total Servings:8 8 servings (about)

Ingredients

7 cups cubed seeded watermelon 1 cup crumbled feta cheese

½ red onion, thinly sliced

½ cup arugula

⅓ cup pine nuts, toasted

⅓ cup chopped fresh parsley

Step 1: Follow the instructions

¼ cup chopped fresh mint

¼ cup olive oil

2 tablespoons fresh lemon juice

½ teaspoon salt ½ teaspoon freshly ground black pepper

Combine watermelon, feta cheese, red onion, arugula, pine nuts, parsley, and mint in a large mixing bowl.

2nd Action

Whisk olive oil, lemon juice, salt, and pepper together in a small bowl; drizzle over salad and toss to coat.

Nutrition Facts Per Serving: 187 calories; protein 5.1g; carbohydrates 12.9g; fat 13.9g; cholesterol 16.7mg; sodium 358.4mg.

Herb Watermelon Feta Salad

This is a delicious summer salad. The ingredients really go well together.

20 minutes to prepare 20 minutes total Servings:12 Yield:12 servings

Ingredients

½ large chilled seedless watermelon, cut into 1-inch cubes 1 small red onion, sliced

1 cup thinly sliced fresh basil leaves 1 cup chopped fresh cilantro

½ cup minced fresh mint leaves 2 limes, juiced 1 (4 ounce) package crumbled feta cheese 3 tablespoons olive oil

2 tablespoons balsamic vinegar, or more to taste To taste, season with salt and black pepper.

Directions

1.

Gently toss watermelon, onion, basil, cilantro, mint, lime juice, feta cheese, olive oil, balsamic vinegar, salt, and black pepper together in a large bowl.

Facts on Nutrition

Per Serving: 177 calories; protein 4g; carbohydrates 31.1g; fat 6g; cholesterol 8.4mg; sodium 111.9mg.

Arugula and Watermelon Salad

An interesting mix of arugula, watermelon, and feta cheese creates one great summer salad!

20 minutes to prepare 20 minutes total Servings:12 Yield:12 servings

Ingredients

2 (5 ounce) packages arugula

½ large watermelon, seeded and cubed 1 red onion, sliced

1 cup crumbled feta cheese

1 ½ cups balsamic vinaigrette

Directions 1.

Toss the arugula, watermelon, red onion, and feta cheese with the balsamic vinaigrette in a large bowl. Serve cold.

Nutrition Facts Per Serving: 245 calories; protein 4.8g; carbohydrates 33.5g; fat 12.4g; cholesterol 11.1mg; sodium 499.9mg.

Conclusion

Blue Zones are areas of the world in which people live exceptionally long lives. Studies have found that genetics only play a 20–30 percent role in longevity. People in Blue Zones typically eat a 95 percent plant-based diet that's rich in legumes, whole grains, vegetables and nuts, all of which can help reduce the risk of death.

Caloric restriction and periodic fasting are common in Blue Zones. Both these practices can significantly reduce risk factors for certain diseases and prolong healthy life.

People in some Blue Zones drink one to two glasses of red wine per day, which may help prevent heart disease and reduce the risk of death.

Moderate physical exercise that is built into daily life, such as walking and climbing stairs, may help prolong life.

People in Blue Zones get sufficient sleep. Seven hours of sleep at night and naps of no more than 30 minutes during the day may help reduce the risk of heart disease and death. Factors other than diet and exercise play an important role in longevity. Religion, life purpose, family and social networks can also influence how long you live.

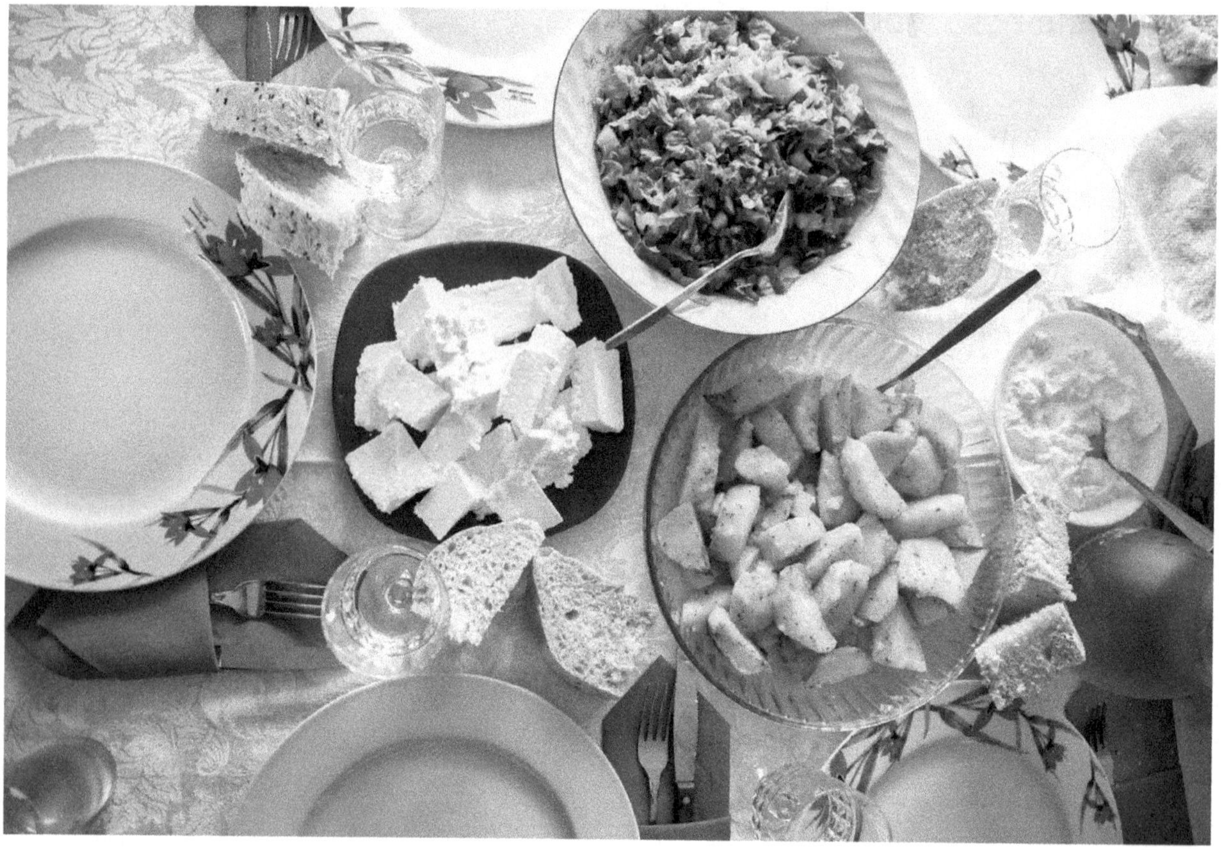

FOOD GUIDELINES

95% plant-based | **5%** animal-based

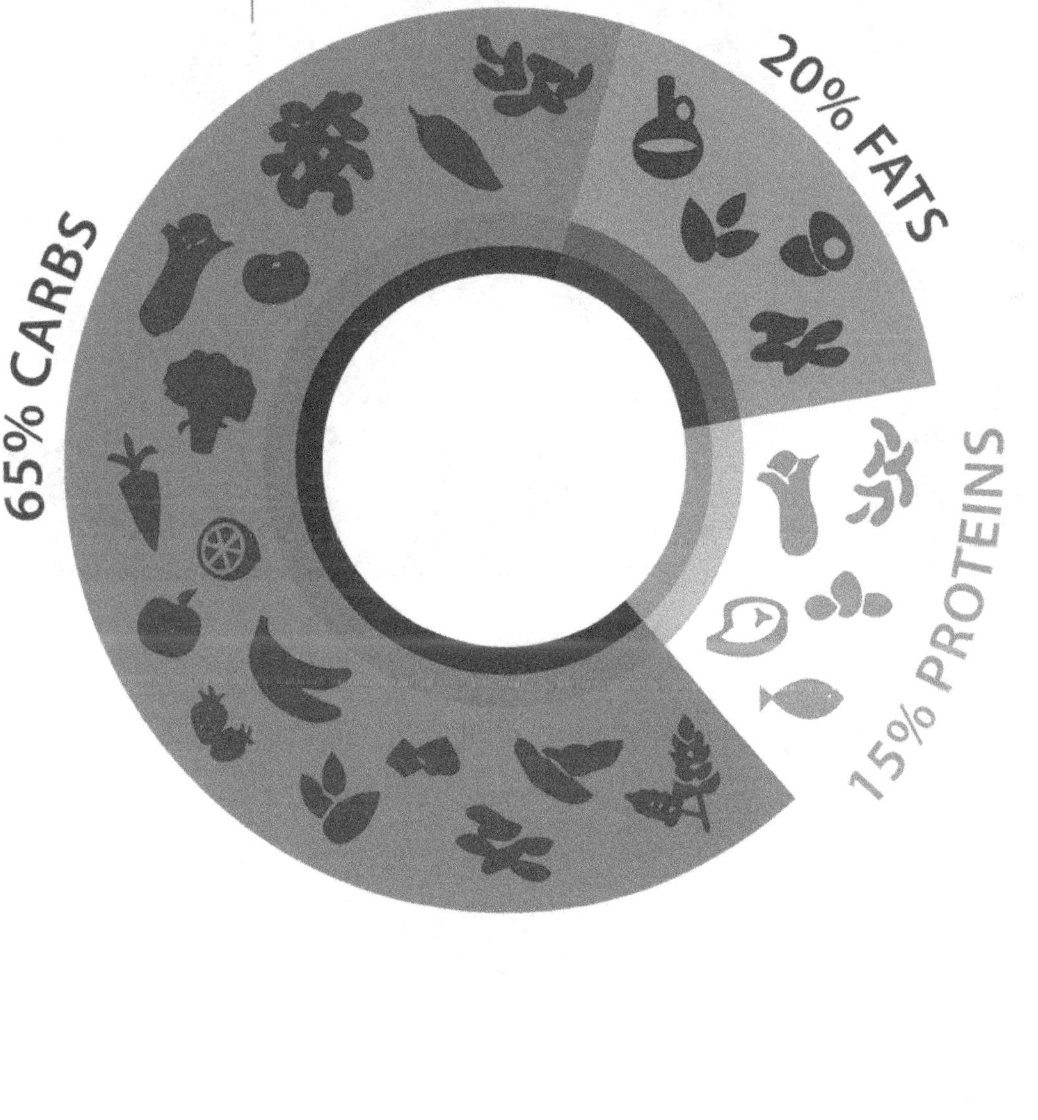

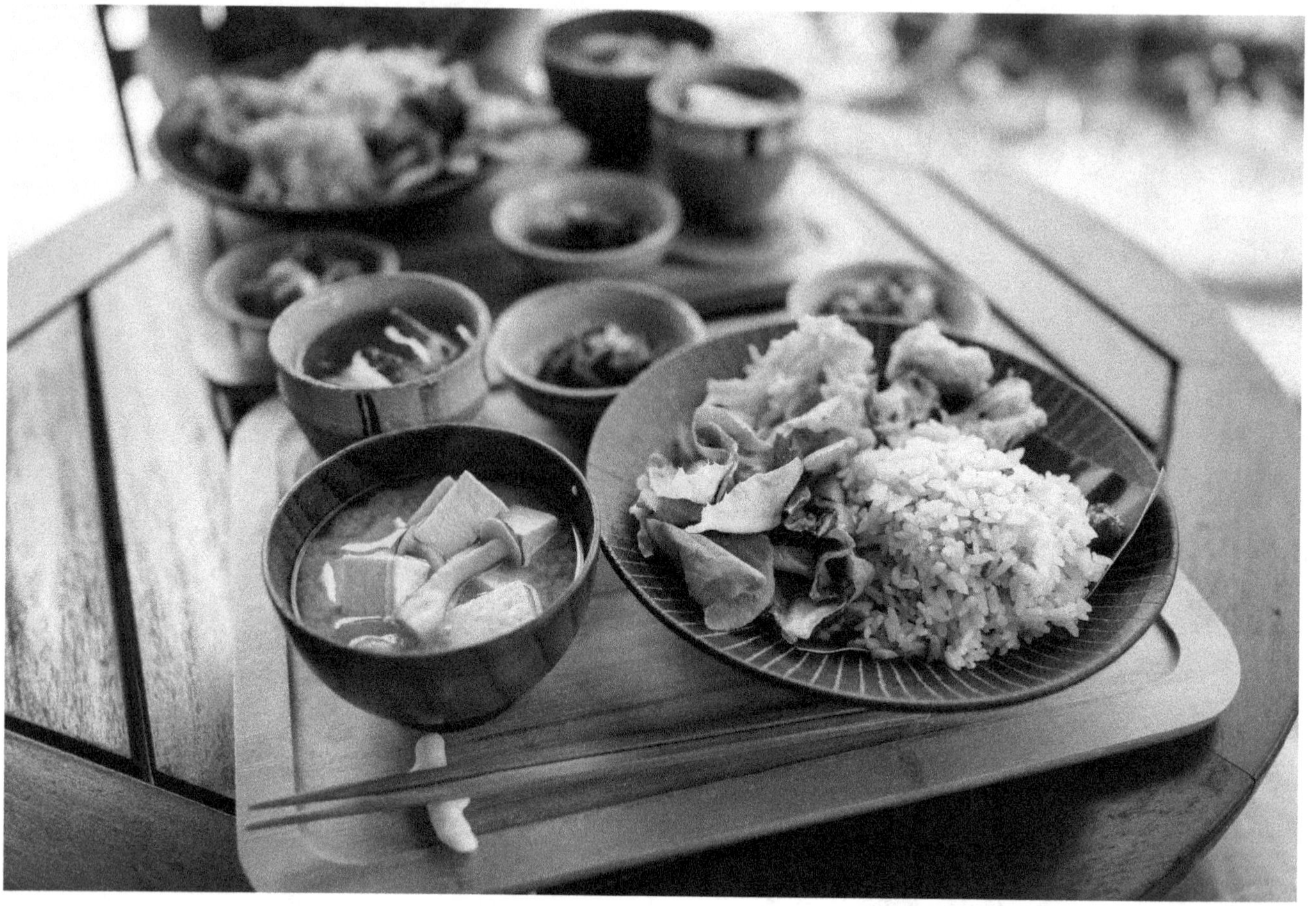

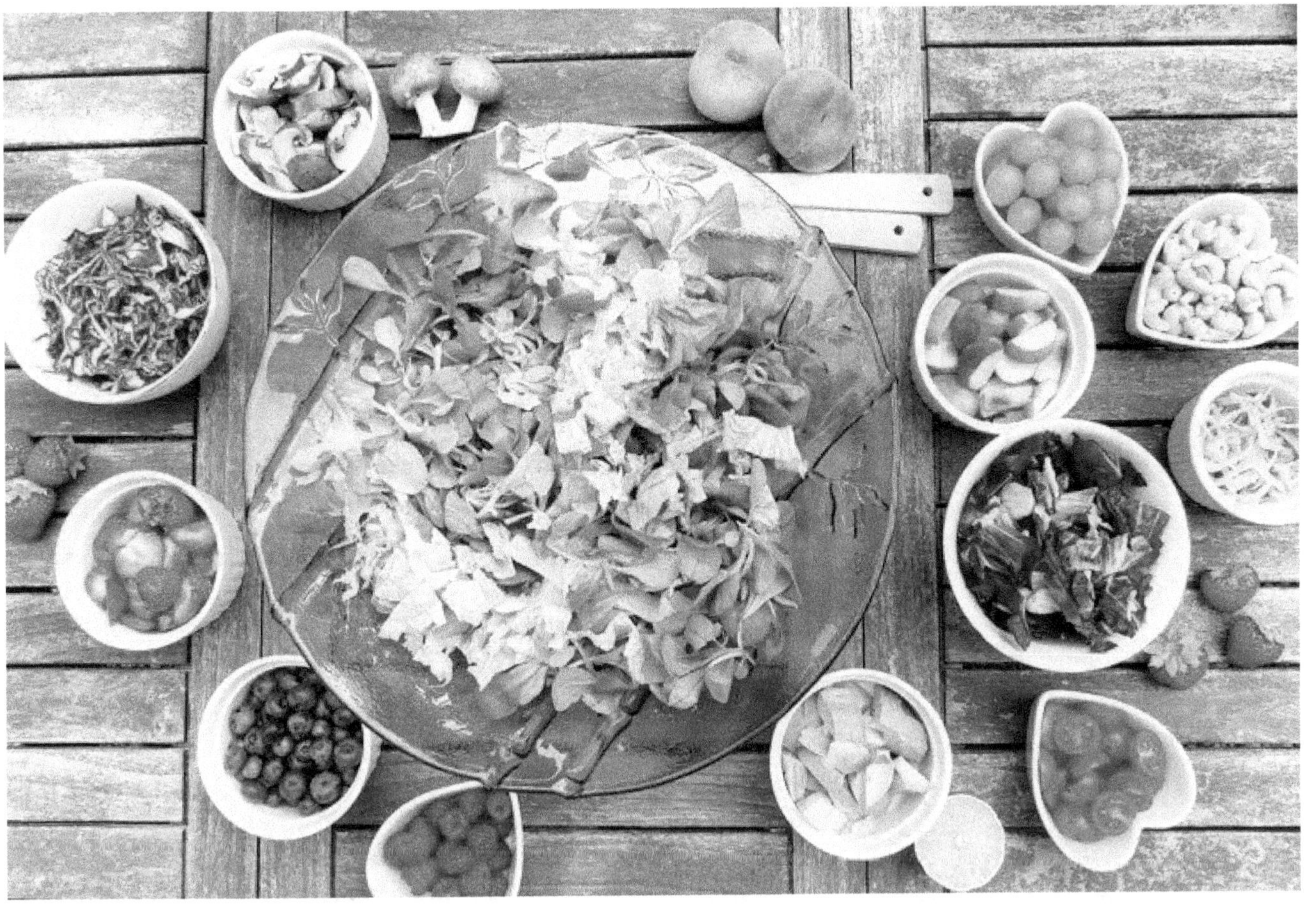

Blue Zones Power 9®

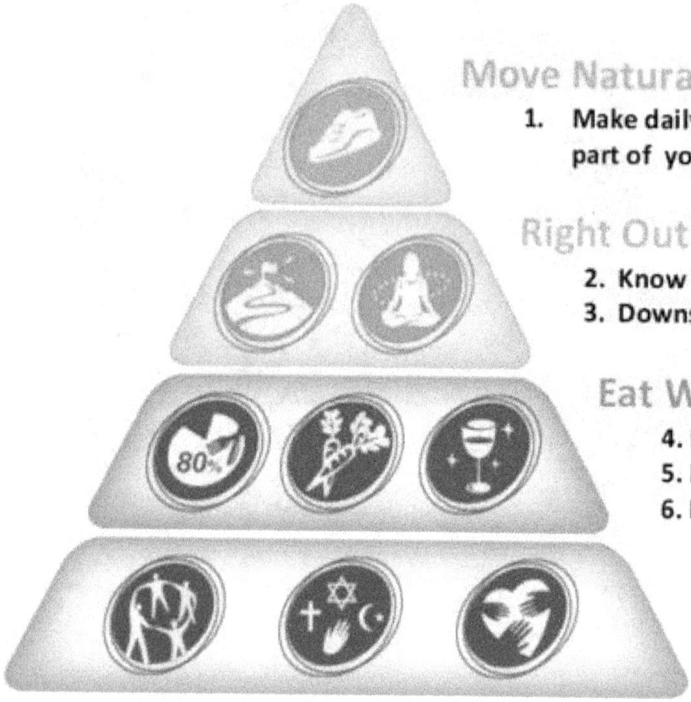

Move Naturally

1. Make daily physical activity an unavoidable part of your environment

Right Outlook

2. Know your purpose
3. Downshift: Work less, slow down, take vacations

Eat Wisely

4. Eat until 80% full
5. More veggies, less meat & processed food
6. Drink a glass of red wine each day

Belong

7. Create a healthy social network
8. Connect/reconnect with religion
9. Prioritize family

CPSIA information can be obtained
at www.ICGtesting.com
Printed in the USA
LVHW060853210122
708837LV00017B/469

9 781804 372289